# A VISIT TO THE HOSPITAL

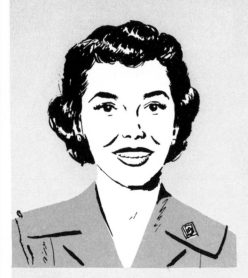
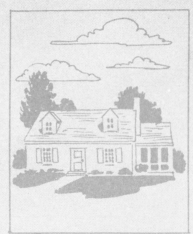
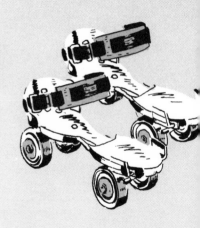
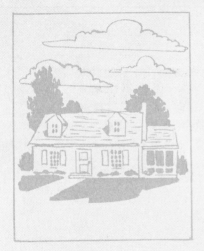
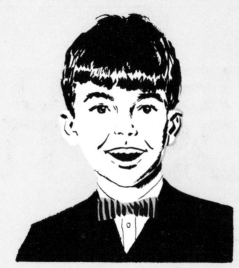
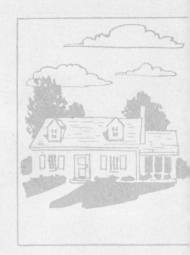
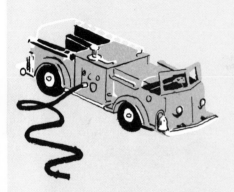
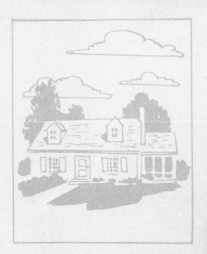
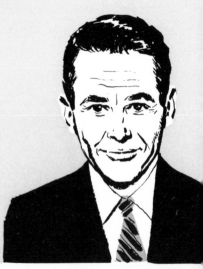

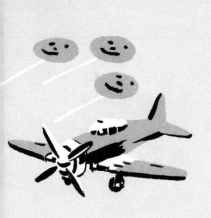
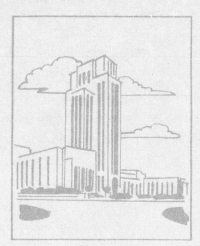
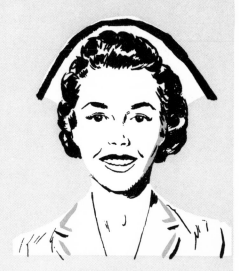
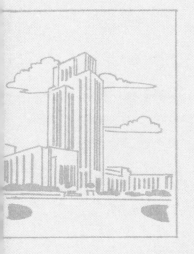
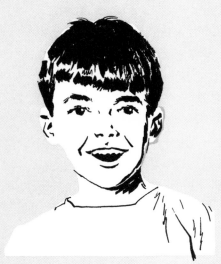
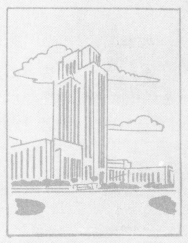
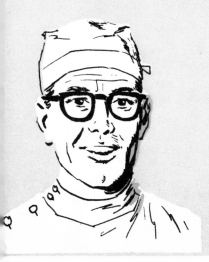
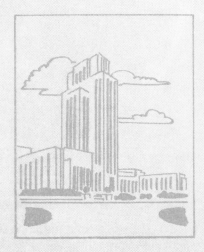
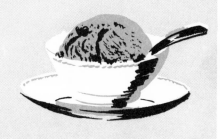

# FOREWORD

If your child is going to have an operation, you can help him have a better hospital experience by telling him ahead of time what to expect. It is the unfamiliar and the unexpected that frightens children. Children who are adequately prepared are actually able to make of their operation a constructive and beneficial experience. Here are some of the things that you as parents, can do to help:

1.  Tell your child the truth. Be forthright and calm when you answer his questions—but, above all, be honest.

2.  Give him the reason for his operation; if it is a tonsillectomy, explain that he will then have fewer colds and more time to play.

3.  Tell him what to expect at the hospital. Avoid surprises and confusion.

4.  Emphasize that separation from his parents is only for a short while—that he will soon return home.

5.  Let him take an active part planning his hospital stay.

6.  Explain that anesthesia is a special way of being fast asleep for a short time, so that he will feel no pain during the operation.

7.  If it is a tonsillectomy, inform him that his throat will hurt after the operation, but that it will feel better with every passing day.

8.  Don't let your child see your own anxiety. If you are worried, he naturally will be, too.

9.  Try to be with him as much as possible at the hospital — overnight if you can.

10. Don't tell your child the exact date of the operation too far in advance.

This book, "A Visit To The Hospital," will serve as a helpful guide to parents. The story was carefully planned to follow a technique, successful in preparing many children for surgery.

*Lester L. Coleman, M. D.*

Associate Attending Surgeon, Manhattan Eye, Ear and Throat Hospital, New York, N.Y.
Vice President, The Academy of Psychosomatic Medicine

# A VISIT TO THE HOSPITAL

Written by *Francine Chase*
Pictures by *James Bama*

Prepared Under the Supervision of
*Lester L. Coleman, M.D.*

With an Introduction by
*Flanders Dunbar, M.D.*

GROSSET & DUNLAP • NEW YORK
**A FILMWAYS COMPANY**

# INTRODUCTION

By Flanders Dunbar, M. D., Med. Sc. D., Ph. D.
Editor-in-Chief, Emeritus, American Psychosomatic Society

Each year, thousands of children all over America enter hospitals for operations. Usually, it is for the removal of tonsils and adenoids, but whether it is for a hernia, eye or any other operation, even an emergency one, the emotional preparation of the child is most important.

Children can be frightened and shocked by contacts with new and unexplained places. Many children are familiar with parks, theaters, libraries and churches in their own towns. But fewer children know about hospitals — and, as with most things about which little is known, hospitals may appear as mysterious and frightening places.

The children who are not frightened are often the ones who have been told ahead of time everything that is about to happen to them. Too frequently, when children are not told why they are going to a hospital, and why they are being separated from their parents, they may become fearful, suspicious and resentful.

Many of these children stay angry and for years, sometimes, remain resentful toward those who took them to the hospital. These children may carry needless scars of unpleasant hospital experiences into adolescence and adulthood.

At times, parents who have themselves been frightened by surgery, have difficulty in explaining a hospital and an operation to their own children.

That is why Dr. Lester L. Coleman had this book prepared. Parents and children who read it will find it easier to understand and talk about the reasons for operations, hospitalization, anesthesia and the brief period away from home.

Physicians, too, will be glad to have the suggestions given to help make a visit to the hospital a growth experience. A little time in thoughtful preparation can add immeasurably to the immediate and future security and happiness of the children who are about to make their first visit to the hospital.

**1977 Printing**
Library of Congress Catalog Card Number: 76-53873
ISBN: 0-448-14011-X
© by Grosset & Dunlap, Inc., 1957

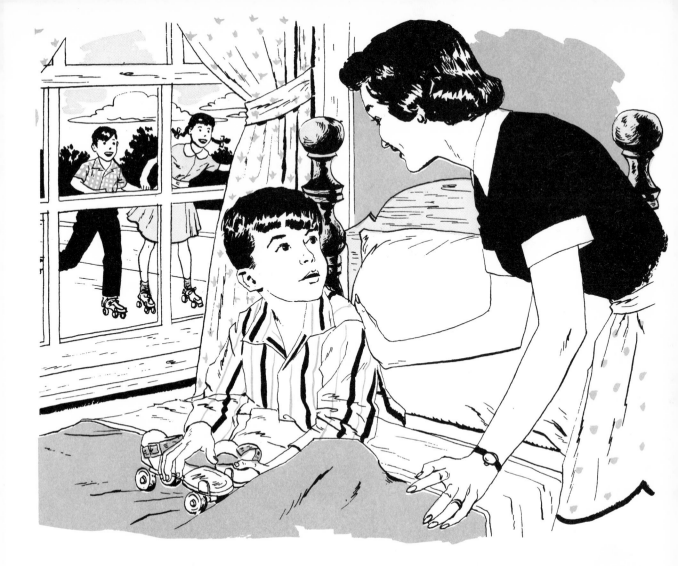

Stevie's friends were outside roller skating. But not Stevie. He was sick in bed again with a cold. It was no fun being in bed while all the other children were outside playing.

Stevie asked his mommy, "Why do I have to have so many colds? I wanted to go skating today with my new ball-bearing skates."

Mommy said, "I know — and I'm sorry. Maybe it's your tonsils that are giving you colds. That often happens."

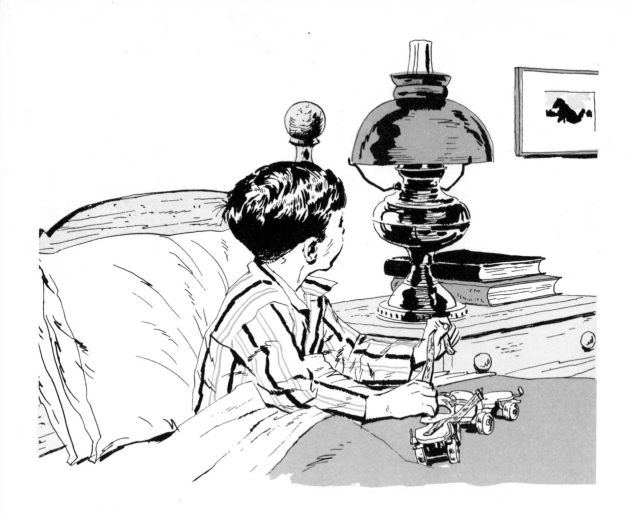

"Tonsils?" Stevie asked. "What are tonsils?"

Mommy said, "Tonsils are two little things in the back of our throats. Everybody is born with them. The funny thing is this. When children are very little, their tonsils help to keep them well. But when children grow older—like you, Stevie— tonsils very often cause colds and sore throats. Then they're not needed any more, so the doctor takes them out."

Stevie asked, "Is it time for my tonsils to come out?"

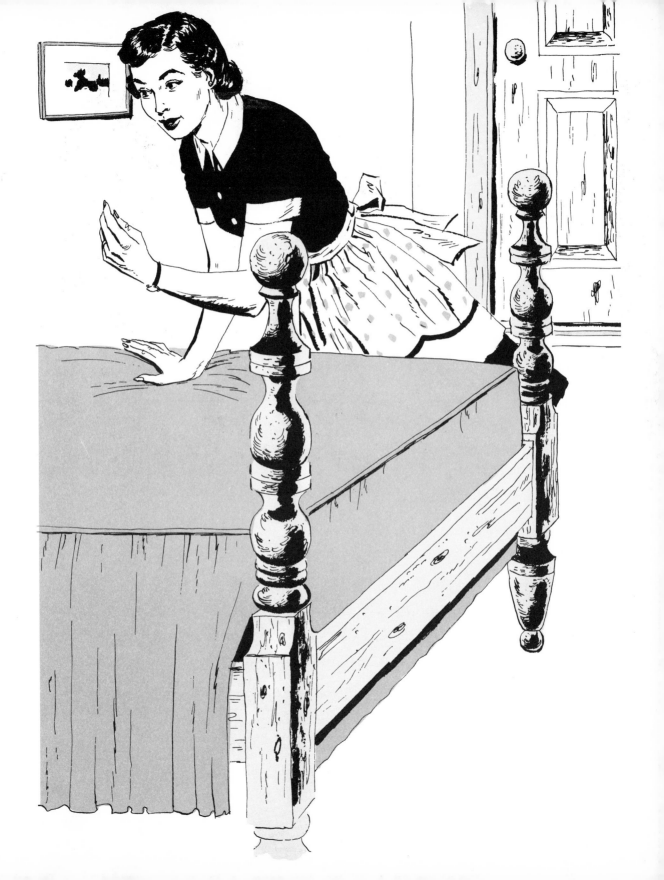

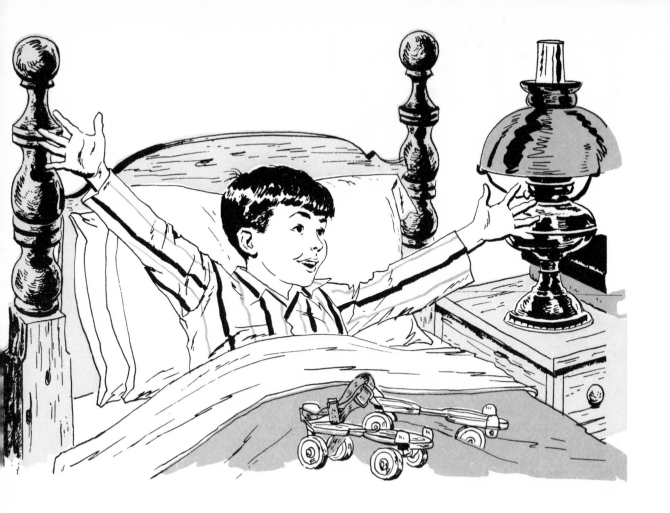

"Well," she said, "we'll have to see the doctor first. He'll tell us if you don't need your tonsils any more."

Stevie said, "I remember when Andy went to the hospital and the doctor took his tonsils out. Andy ate five dishes of ice cream in one day!" Andy was Stevie's big brother.

Mommy smiled. "Could you eat that much ice cream?"

"I could eat a thousand million dishes of ice cream!" Stevie shouted. His eyes brightened at the very thought.

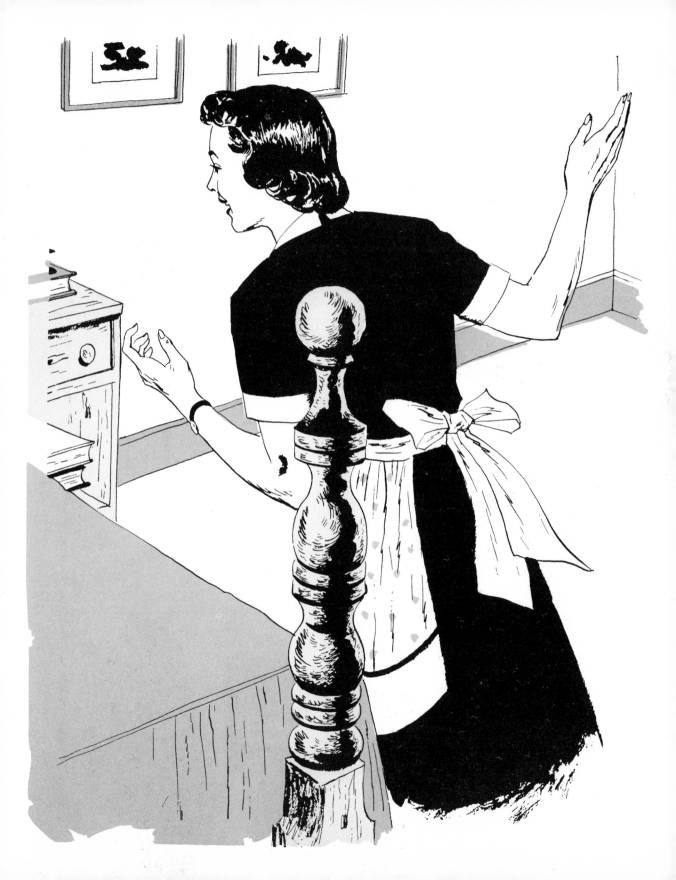

When Stevie was well again, he and his mother took a bus ride to the doctor's office. She let him drop the coins for their fare into the slot. He liked to hear the little bell ring when the money went in. He found a seat by the window. There was so much to see outside that he didn't want to miss a thing.

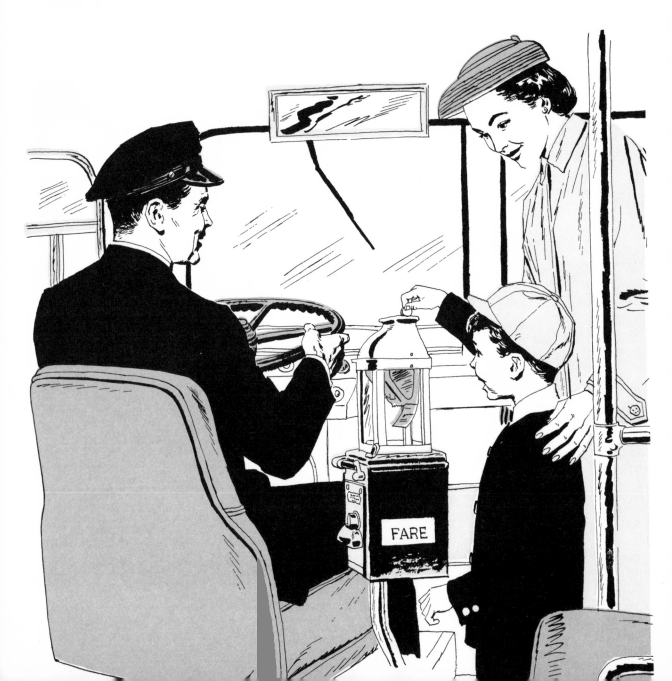

FARE

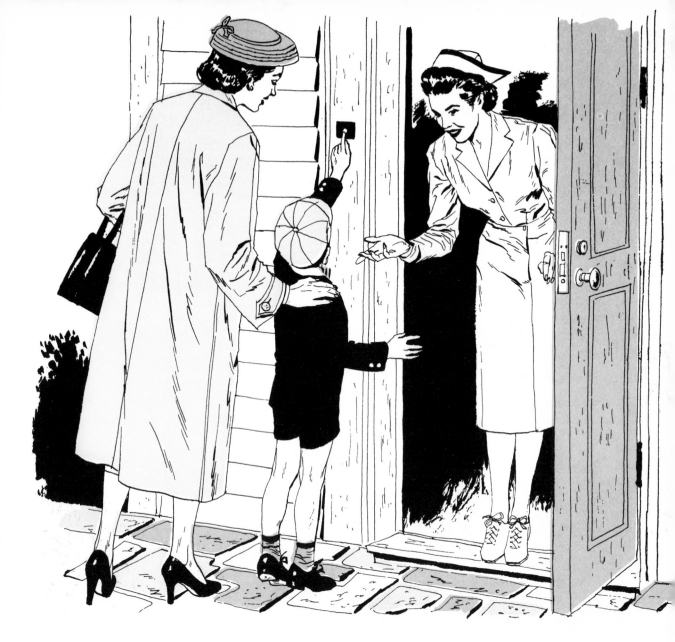

Soon they arrived at the doctor's office. Stevie was tall enough to reach the doorbell, and he pressed it hard. The doctor's nurse greeted them at the door.

"Hello, Stevie," she said. "The doctor will be so glad to see you!"

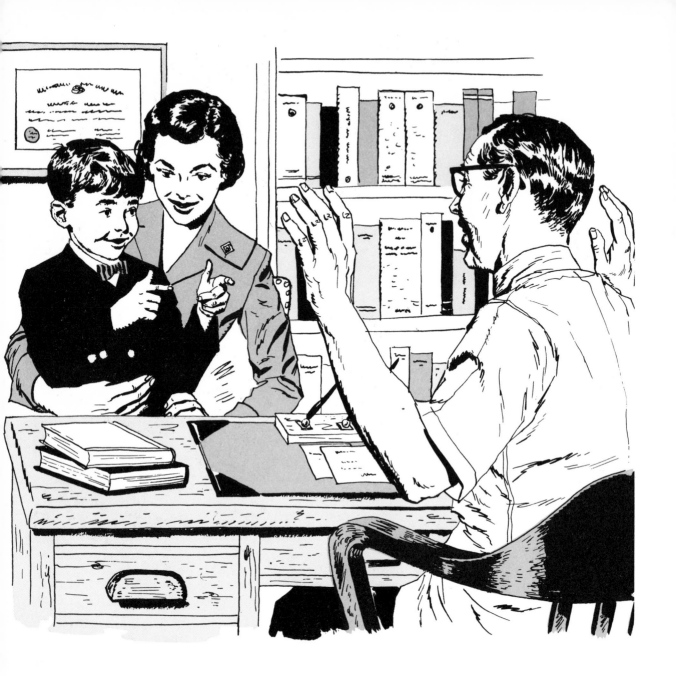

"Hi, Stevie," the doctor called out. "Come on in. I've been expecting you." Stevie sat down with his mother near the doctor's big desk. They talked about many things, especially about their favorite television programs.

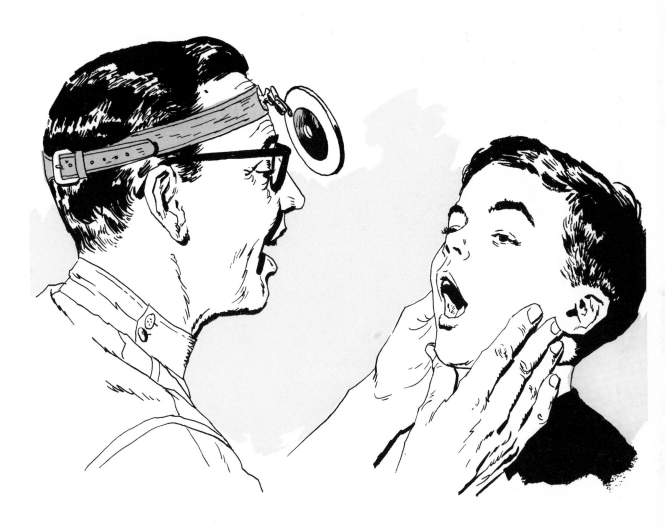

Then the doctor said, "Well, Stevie, your mother tells me
that you've been having lots of sore throats and colds lately.
Let me take a look at your throat and see how I can help you."

Stevie opened his mouth wide.

"Well," said the doctor, "just as I thought. It's those tonsils,
all right. That's why you've been sick in bed so much. They'll
have to come out."

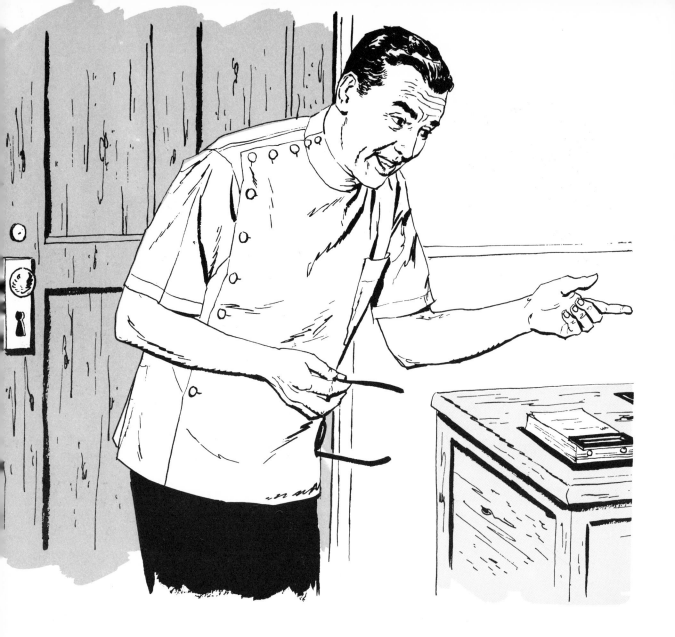

The doctor and Mommy decided that next Tuesday would be a good day to take out the tonsils.

Stevie wasn't too sure he liked this. But after he asked some questions he felt better, because the doctor explained everything so nicely.

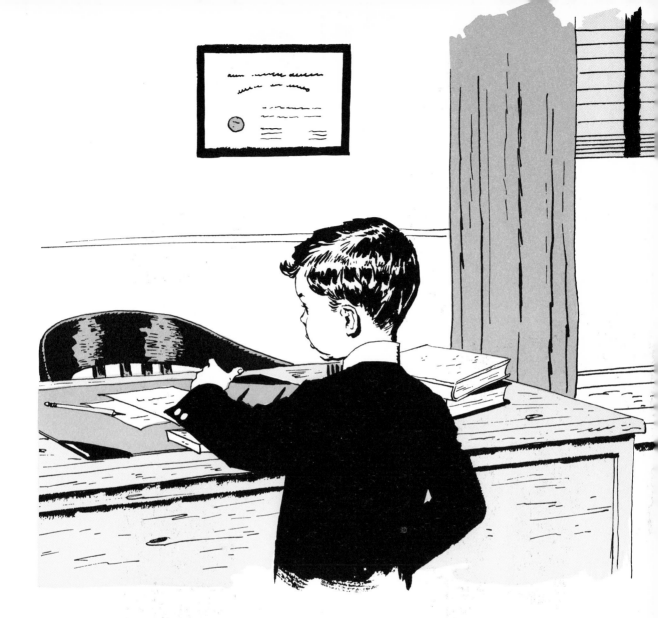

Stevie liked his doctor. He was so friendly and he said things that made him laugh. Stevie said, "When I grow up I'm going to be a doctor—or maybe a cowboy—but I think a doctor."

"I hope you'll be a doctor. Then you can be my assistant," the doctor said.

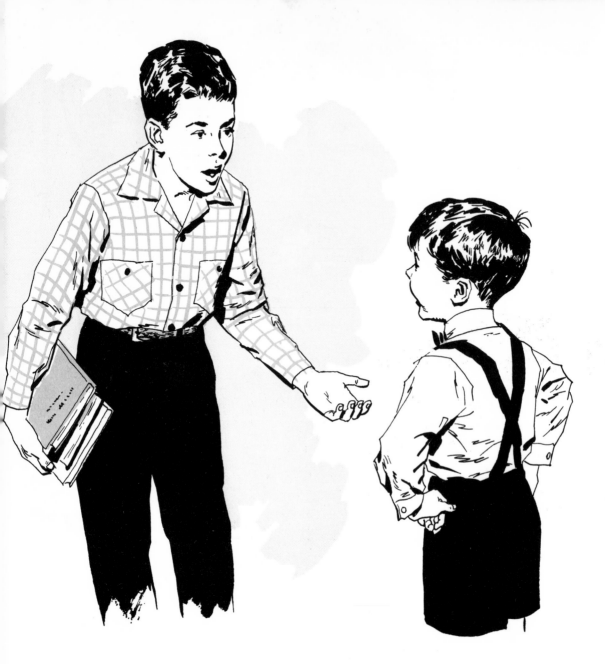

Stevie and Mommy went home. His big brother Andy had
just come home from school.

"What did the doctor say?" Andy asked.

Stevie told him, "He said he's going to take my tonsils out."

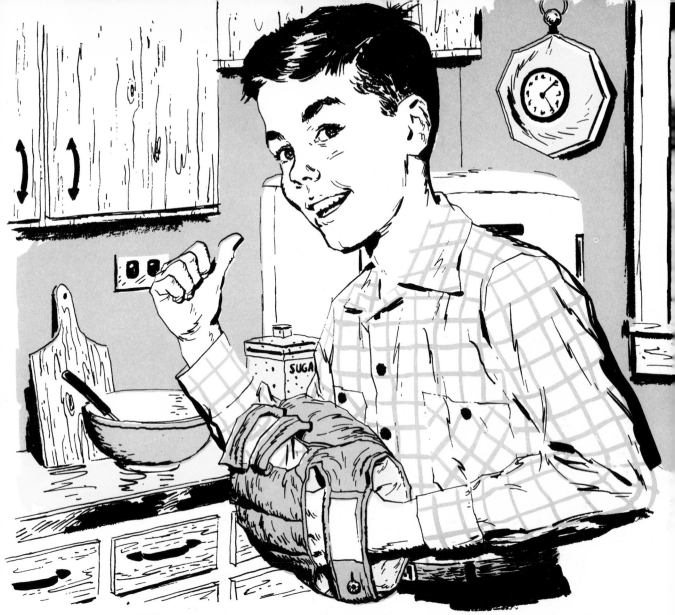

Mommy went into the kitchen to get some chocolate brownies and milk.

Andy and Stevie drank their milk, and ate every crumb of their brownies.

"Come on, Stevie," Andy said to his brother. "Let's go outside and play catch."

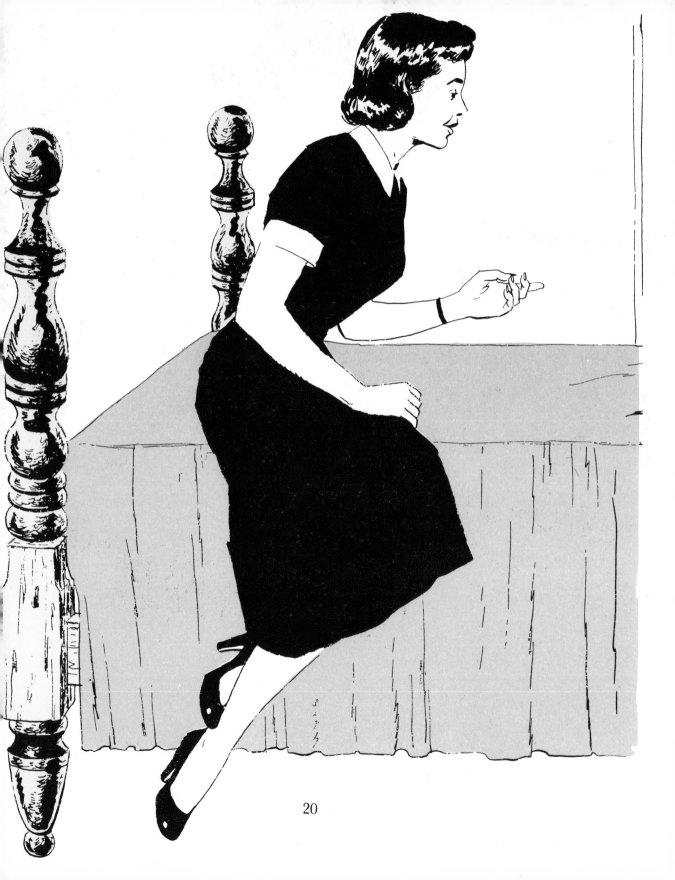

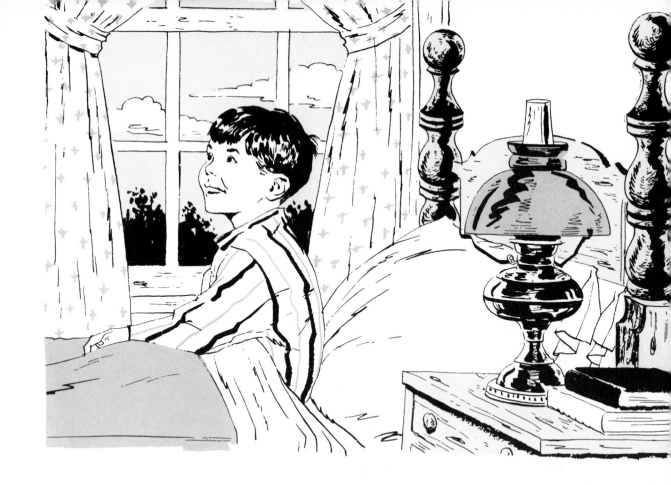

That night when he was going to bed, Stevie asked his mother, "How long will I have to stay at the hospital?"

"Only one day and one night," Mommy answered. She could tell that Stevie was worried about the operation. Then she said, "I'm going to tell you all about the hospital. If you know exactly what's going to happen there, you won't be afraid."

And she did. She told Stevie all about the tonsil operation, and she told him that Mommy or Daddy or maybe both would be with him at the hospital. This made Stevie feel much better.

When Tuesday morning came, Stevie awoke bright and early. He packed his own suitcase. Into it he put his bathrobe, slippers, and favorite books. He took along his own special sleep toy. It wasn't really a toy. It was just an old piece of baby blanket that he loved to sleep with.

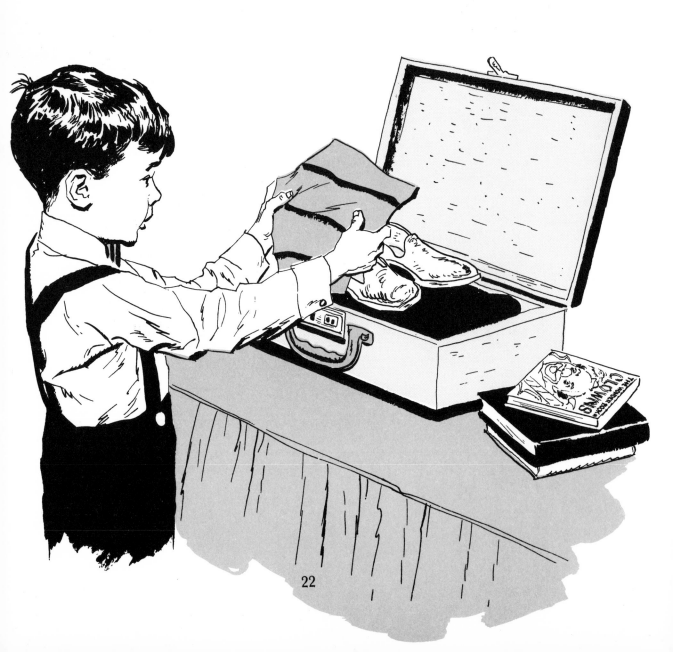

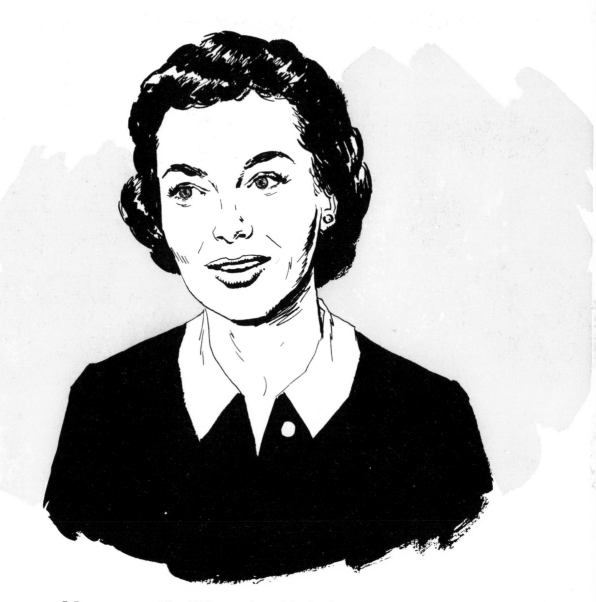

Mommy said, "You shouldn't have breakfast today because the doctor says that if you don't eat just before you have your tonsils out, you'll feel better afterward."

He was too excited to care about breakfast anyway. He wasn't even hungry.

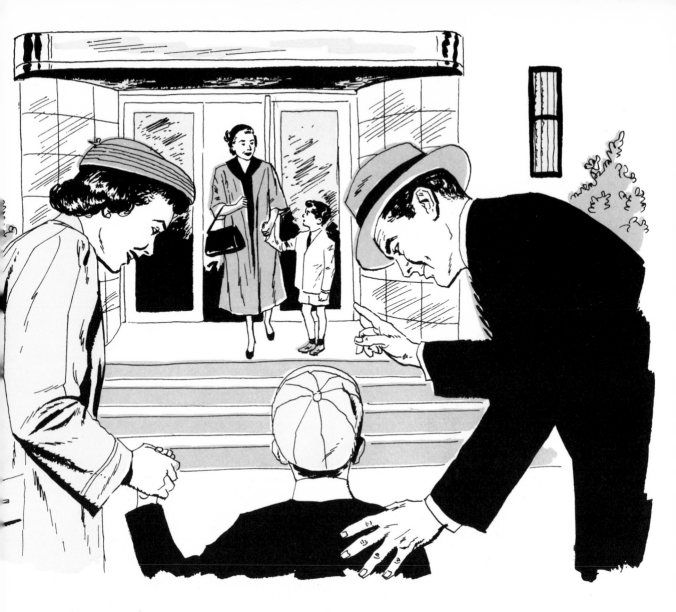

When Stevie and his mother and father got to the hospital, they saw a little boy coming out with his mother.

"I'll bet he had his tonsils out yesterday," said his daddy. "That's why he's going home today."

"And I'll be going home tomorrow!" said Stevie.

"You certainly will," answered Mommy.

Inside the hospital, there were ladies dressed in white who were very busy. One of them smiled at Stevie.

Mommy told him that these ladies were nurses. They were there to help the doctors and to make the children more com-fortable during their stay.

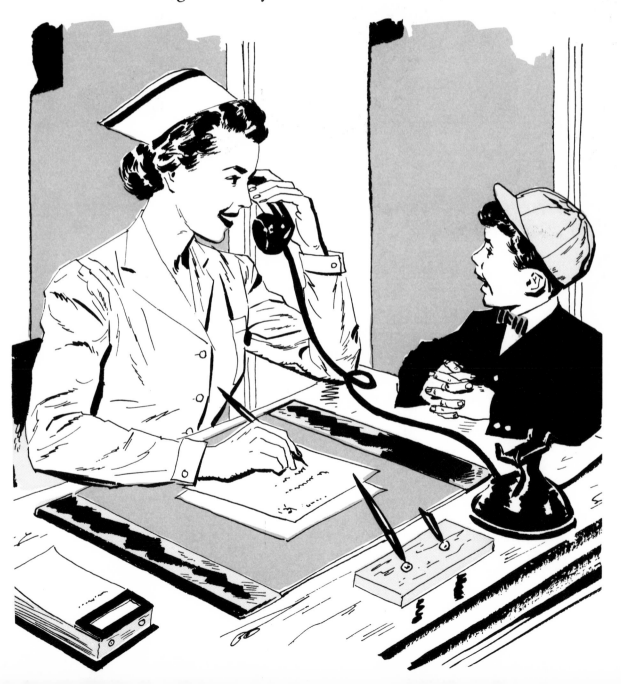

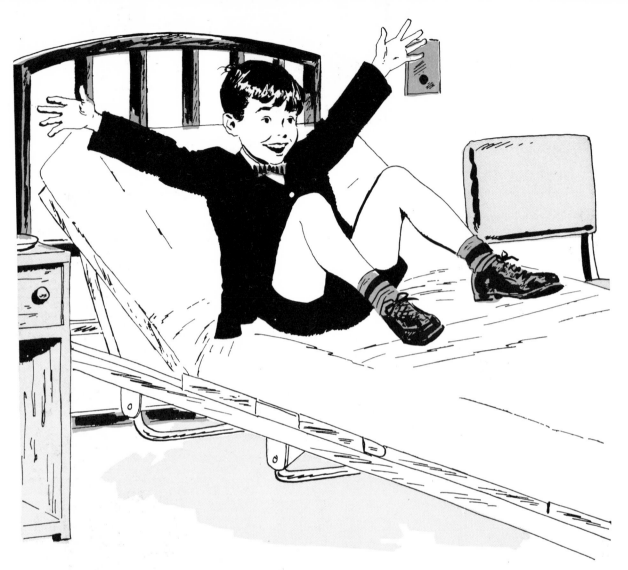

Then they all went up to Stevie's hospital room. Stevie ran over to the bed. He had never seen a hospital bed before. He had fun turning the two handles at the end of the bed. When he turned one handle one way, the top of the bed went up. When he turned it the other way, it went down. Then he turned the other handle. This time it was the bottom of the bed that went up and down.

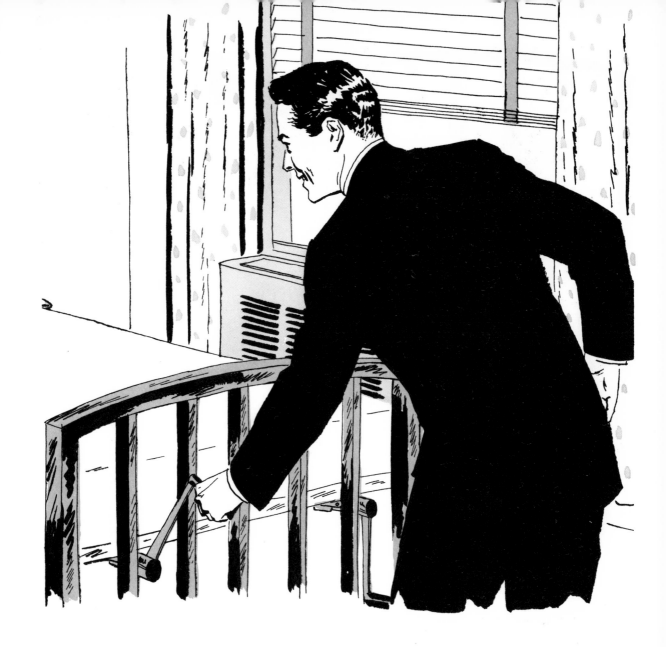

He hopped onto the bed and his daddy made the bed go up and down with him on it.

"Why can't we have beds like this at home?" Stevie giggled. "This is fun!"

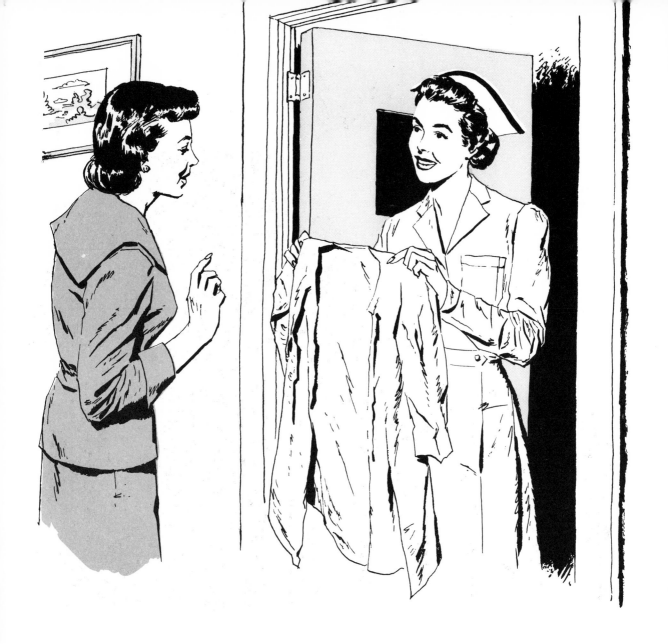

In a few minutes the door opened and a nurse walked in. She gave Mommy a little white jacket and said, "This is for Stevie to put on. It looks like the one his doctor will wear in the operating room."

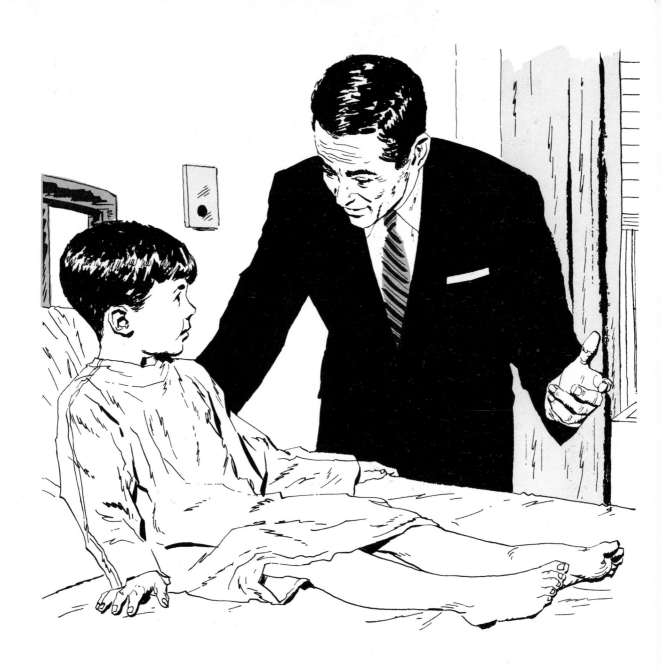

Daddy helped Stevie take off his pants and shirt and put on the jacket. He looked at him and said, "Well, hello, Doctor Stevie! You really do look like a doctor now."

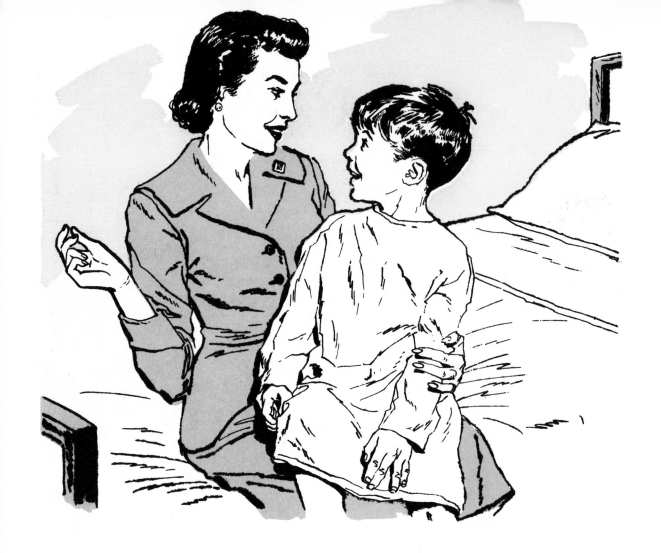

Stevie sat in his mother's lap for a few minutes. She told him that while he was upstairs in the operating room having his tonsils taken out, she and Daddy would be sitting in his room, waiting for him to come back.

"Will I be there very long?" he asked.

"No, it takes only a little while," Mommy answered, "about as long as it takes us to walk to the playground and back to the house again."

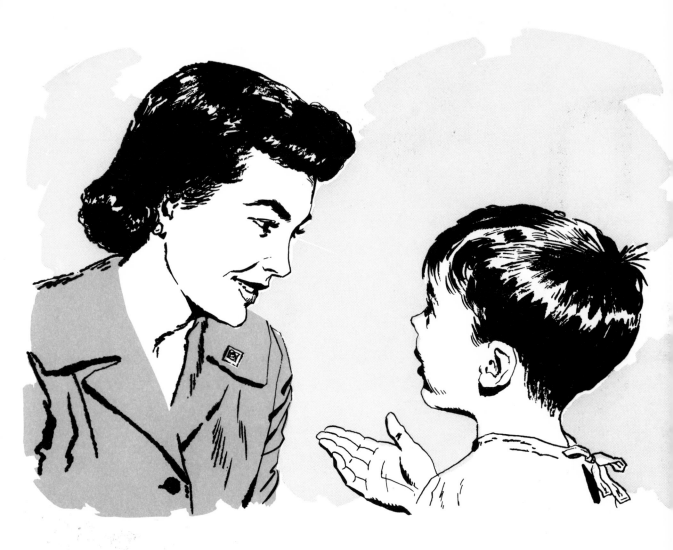

"Why can't you be with me in the operating room?" he **asked** his mother.

"Because only doctors and nurses are **allowed in the operating** room."

"**Will** it hurt?"

"**No,**" Mommy said. "Remember, I told **you that** you won't **feel anything**—because you'll be fast asleep."

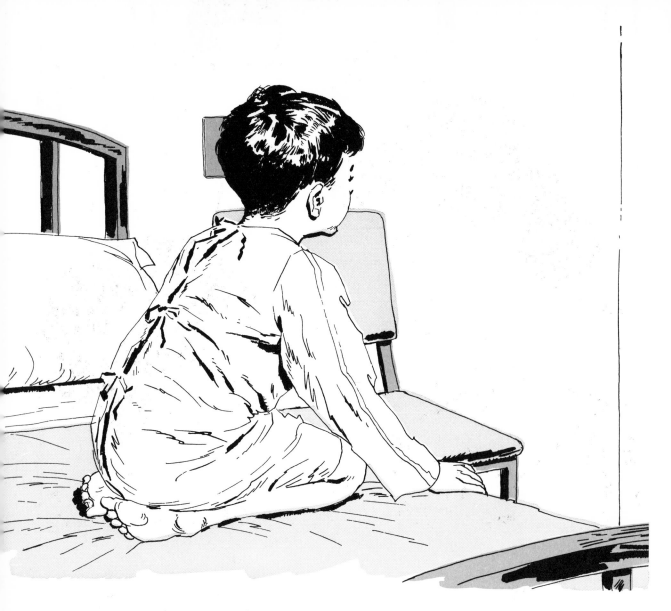

"Why do I have to go to sleep?"

"When children have a tonsil operation," Mommy explained again, "the doctor helps them go to sleep so that they won't feel any pain. In fact, you'll be so fast asleep you won't even know that he is taking out your tonsils."

"How does he do that?" Stevie asked.

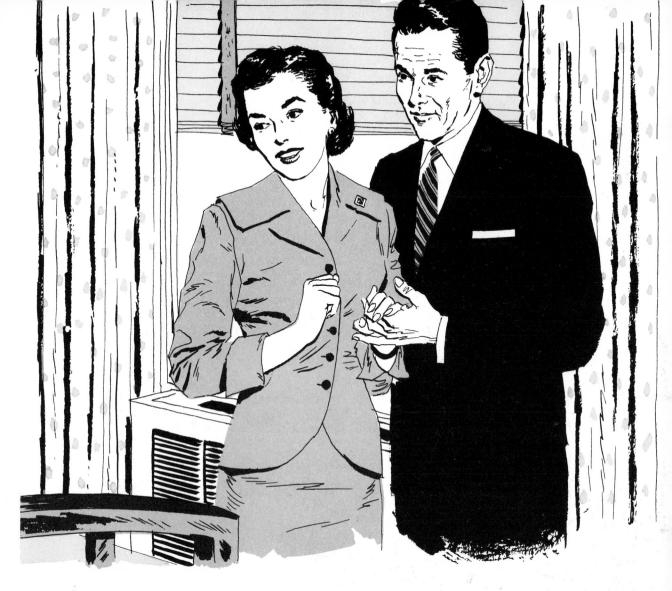

"The doctor will let you blow into something that looks like a balloon. It has a funny smell—something like my nail polish. After you take a few big breaths, you'll fall fast asleep. Then the doctor will take your tonsils out. While you're still sleeping, they'll bring you back to this room and we'll be waiting right here for you.

"When you wake up your throat will feel sore, but every day it will get better and better. And when you get home you may have all the ice cream and soda pop you like, because that will help make your throat feel good."

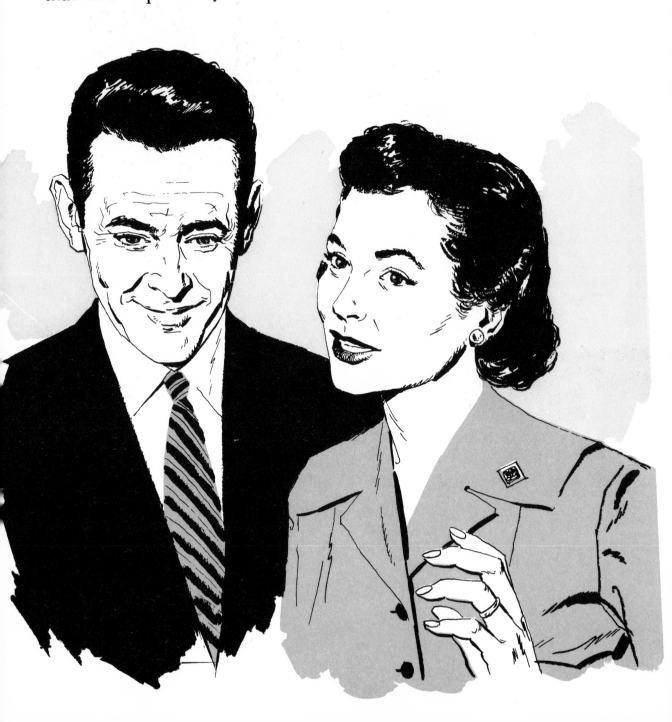

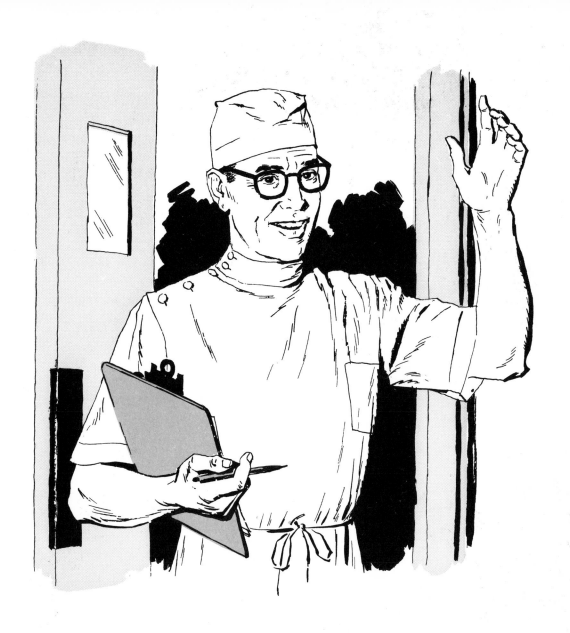

Very soon the door opened and the doctor walked in. He was wearing a white jacket, just like Stevie's.

"Hi, there, Stevie," he said. "It's time to get started." Then the doctor said to Stevie's mother and father, "We'll be right back. So you stay here and wait for us."

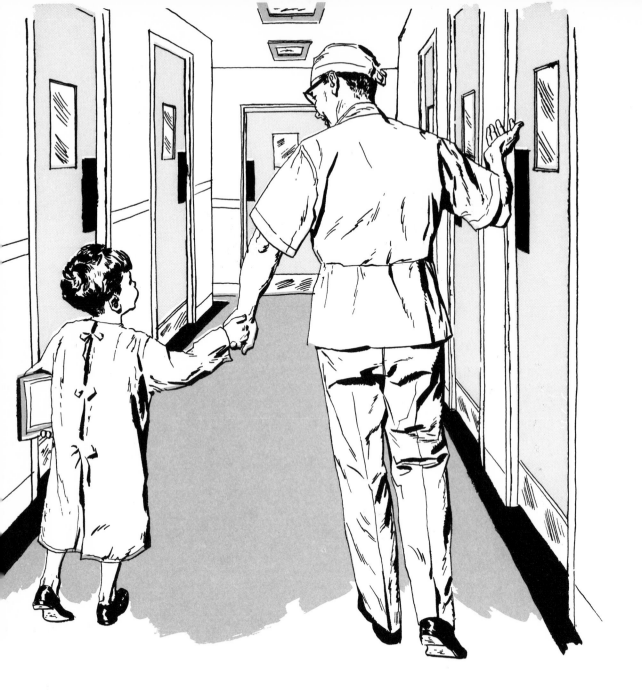

Off they went together to the operating room. While they walked down the hall they had lots of fun making believe that Stevie was the doctor's assistant.

When they got to the operating room, the doctor sat Stevie on the table. Stevie looked around and saw that everything in the room was as white as a new snowfall.

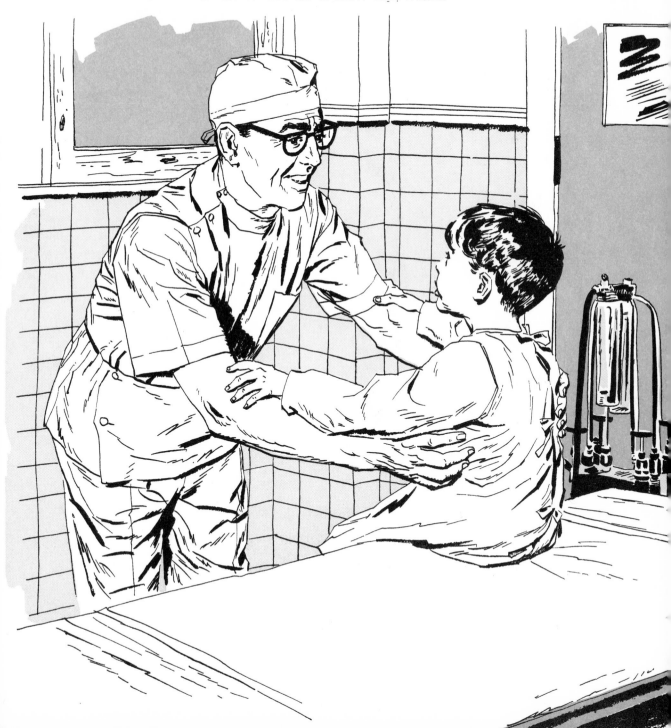

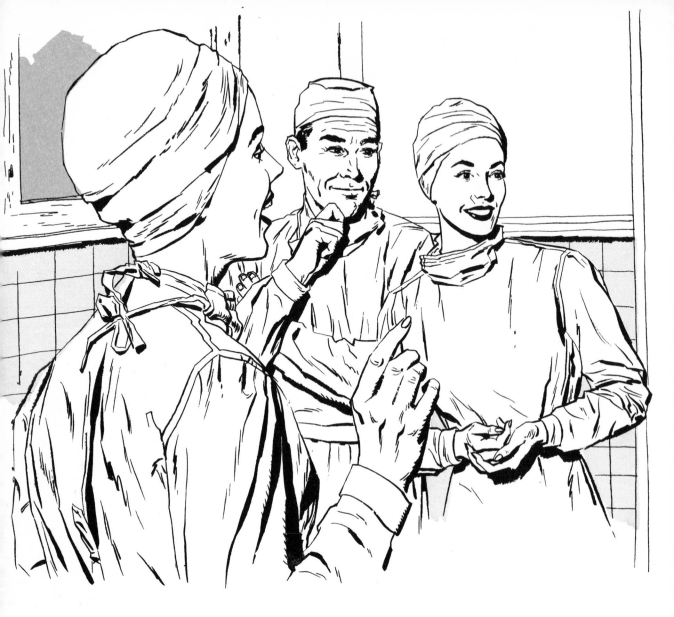

The doctor said, "We use white for the color of our operating room because it looks so sparkling clean."

There were other doctors and nurses in the room. They were all there to help Stevie's doctor. They were wearing white, too.

"Hello, Stevie," said one of the nurses.

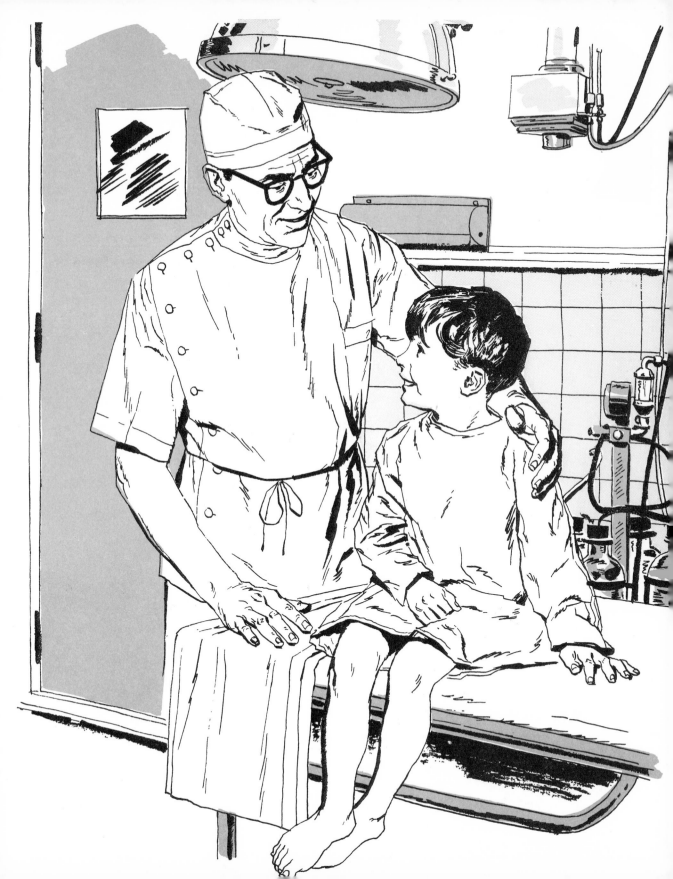

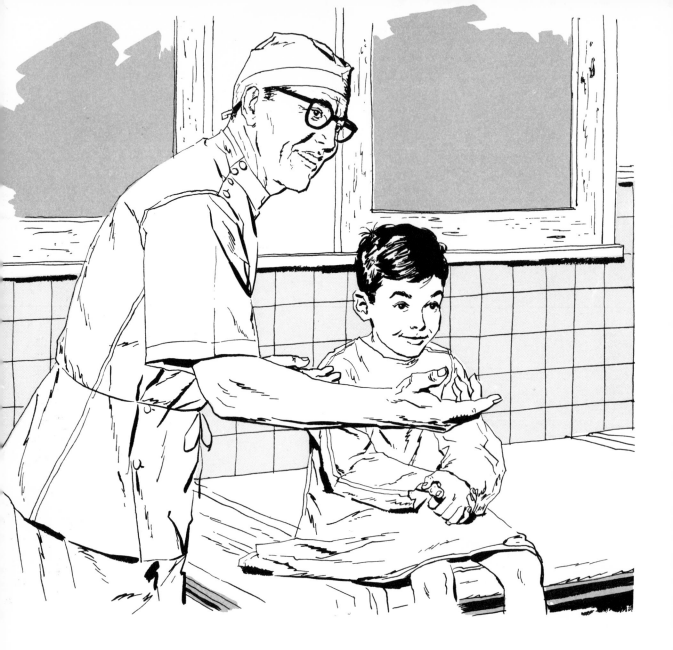

Then the nurse put a little mask over her nose and mouth.
So did the other people.

The doctor said, "Don't they look funny with masks on?
We all have to wear a mask. Because if any of us has a cold,
you won't catch it when our noses and mouths are covered."

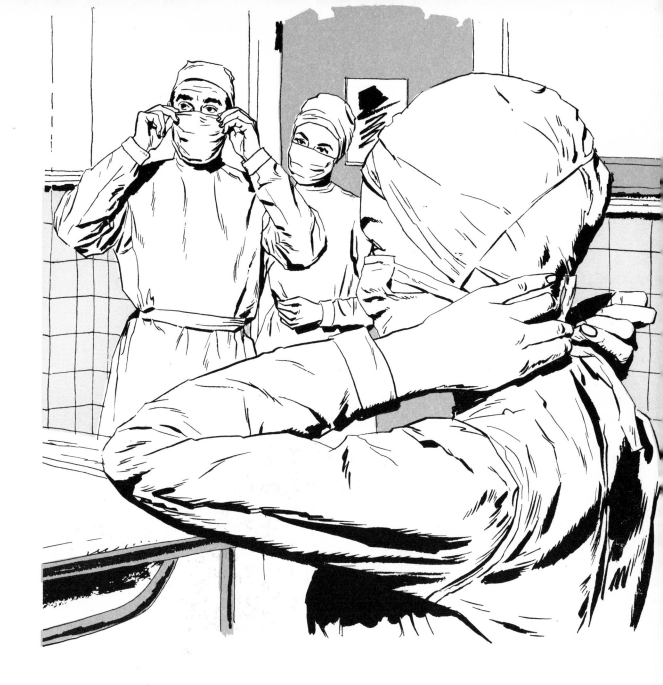

The doctor asked Stevie to lie down so that he could take
out his tonsils. The quicker they were out, the quicker Stevie
could go back to his mommy and daddy.

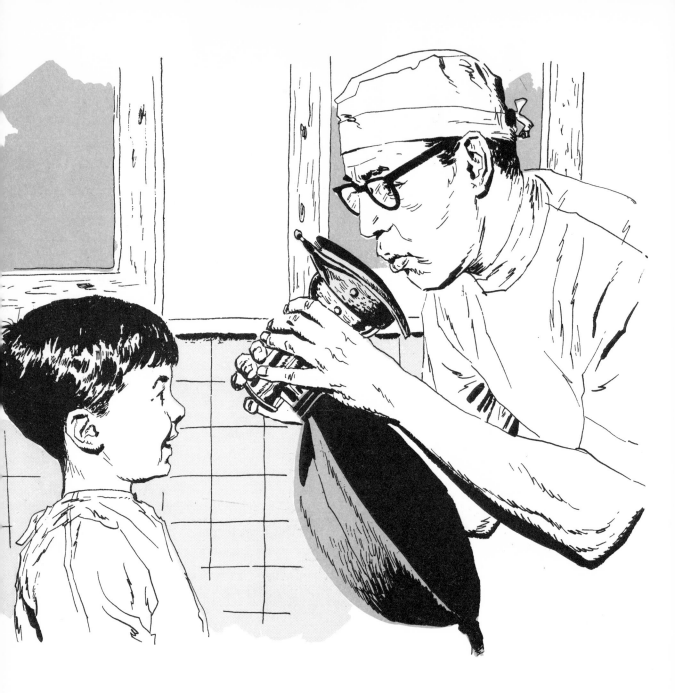

"Now just pretend that you're going to blow up this balloon," the doctor said. "This is the way to do it." He showed him how.

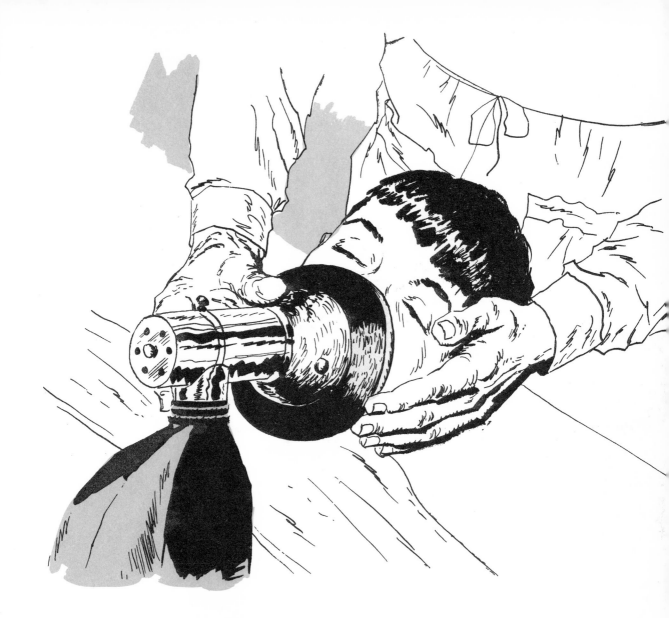

"Now you do it, Stevie. Take a good, deep breath, blow into the balloon, and count to ten."

The balloon smelled funny, just as Mommy had said it would. But Stevie took a good, deep breath and began to count. "One...two...three...four...five...six..." and before he got to seven, he was asleep.

The doctor waited until Stevie was fast asleep. Then he quickly took out the tonsils. It didn't hurt Stevie at all, of course, because the doctor let him stay asleep until the tonsil operation was all over.

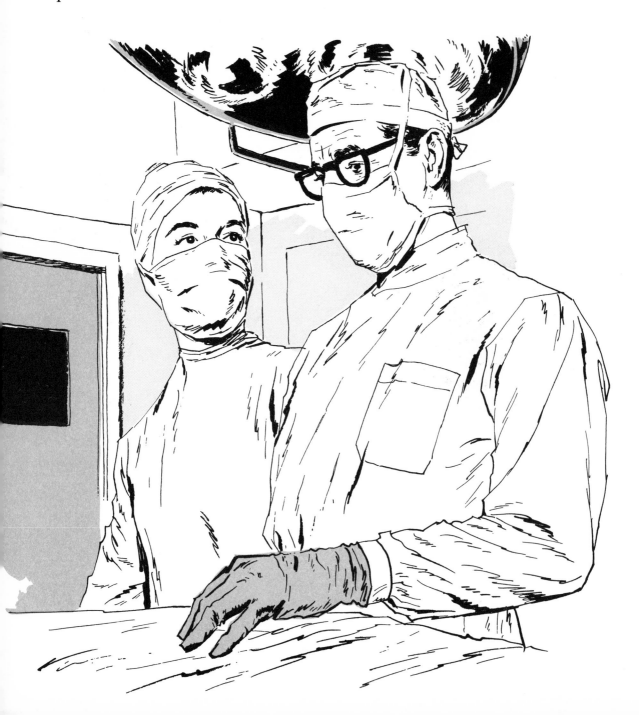

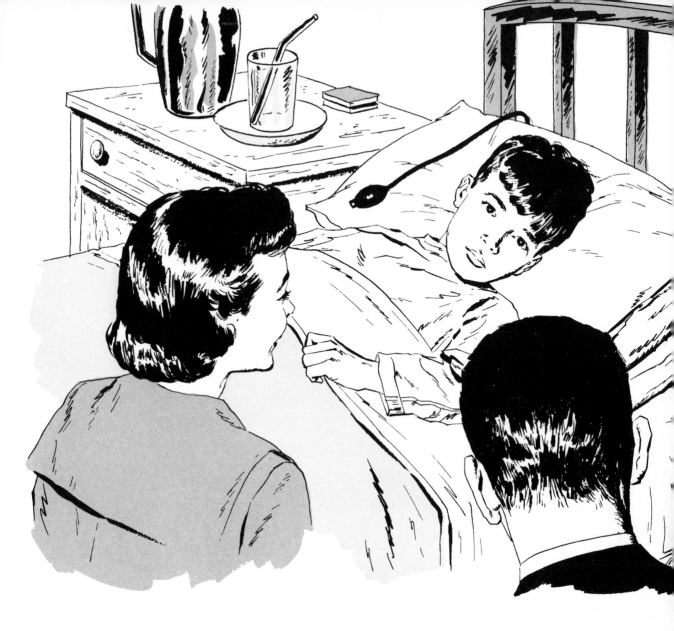

When Stevie woke up, he was already back in his own hospital room. His mommy and daddy were there, too.

"When are my tonsils coming out?" Stevie asked.

"Why, they're already out!" Mommy said.

"My throat hurts," said Stevie.

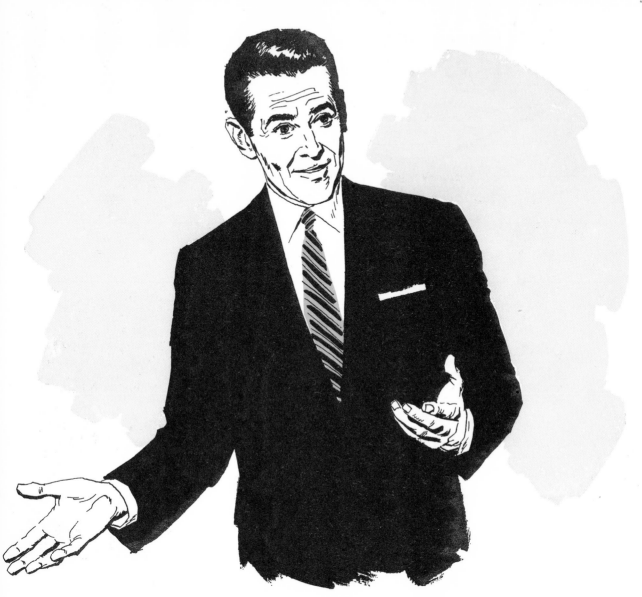

"Yes, son," said his daddy. "We told you your throat would be sore after the operation. But it's going to feel better and better every day. Then you won't have so many sore throats any more. That's why we're all so happy that you had your tonsils taken out. The doctor told us that you were a wonderful patient!"

Stevie dozed off for a nap. When he woke up he drank some cool soda pop. That felt good.

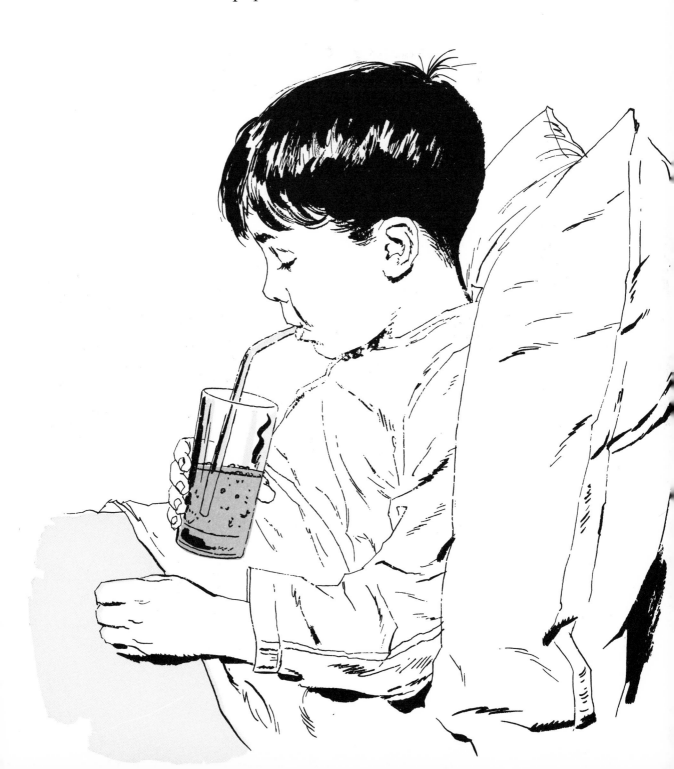

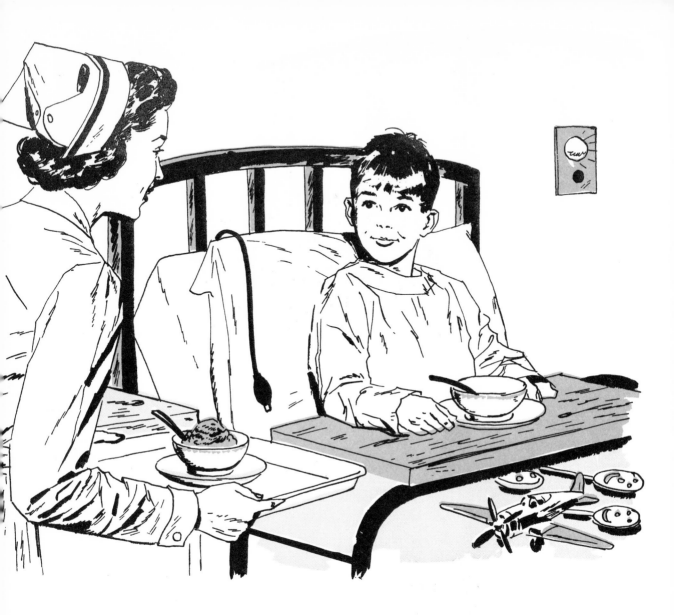

Daddy had surprised Stevie with a new toy—a silvery air-plane that could fly all over the room. His brother Andy had sent him lollipops. And the nurse brought him ice cream. It did make his throat feel better, but he certainly didn't feel like eating a thousand million dishes of ice cream!

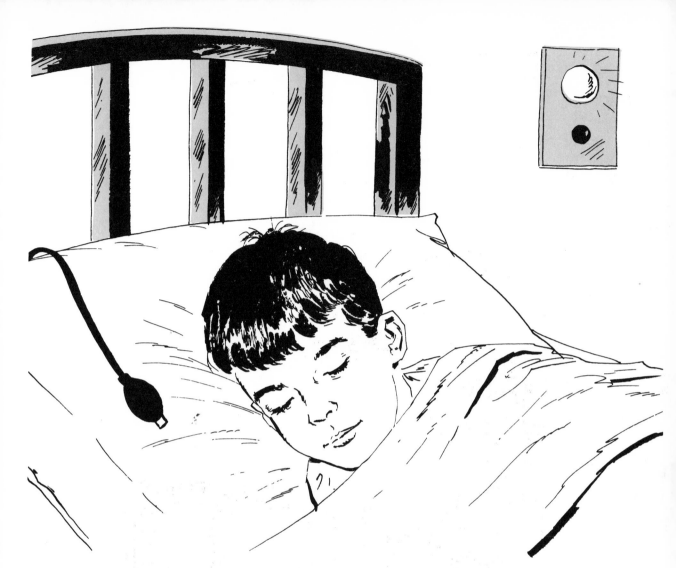

That night he had a good night's sleep in the hospital. There was a little light that was left on in his room so he could see the push button near his bed. The nurse had told Stevie that if he needed anything during the night, all he had to do was push the button. That would ring a bell outside and she would come right in. But Stevie didn't use it at all. In fact, he slept so well that he didn't even hear the nurse come in to see if he was comfortable.

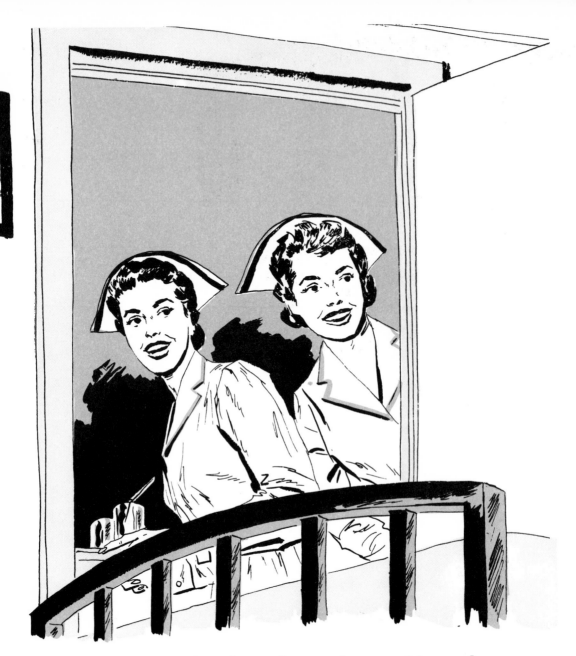

The next morning, when he woke up, he saw his mother
in the room.

"It's time to go home, dear," she said.

She helped Stevie get dressed. They said good-by to the
nurses and were on their way.

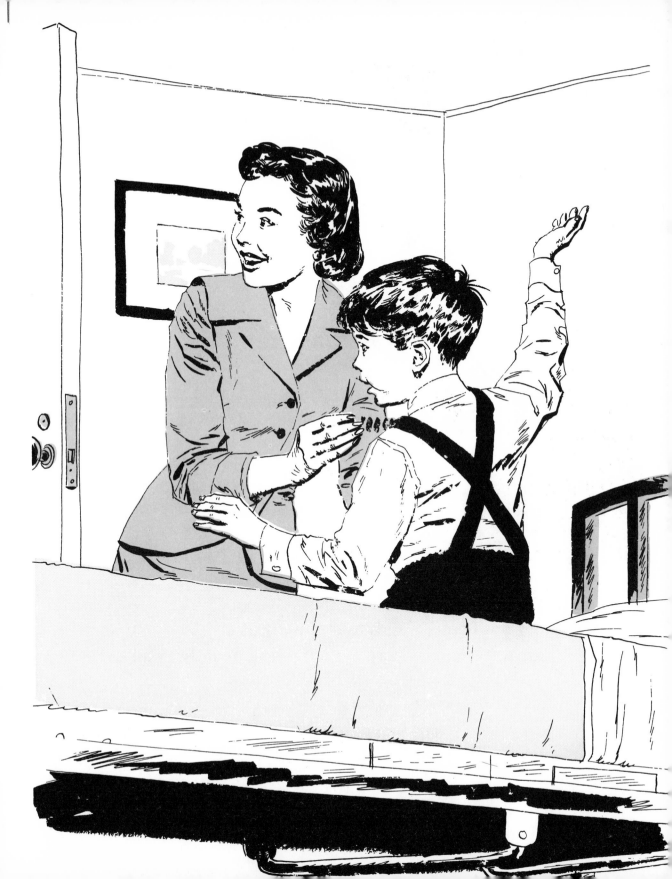

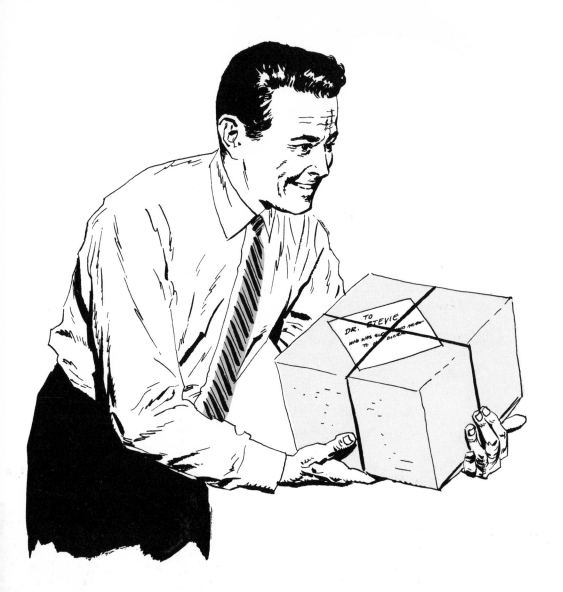

When they got home, Daddy was waiting in the bedroom
with a package in his hand. There was a big card on it that said:

TO

# DR. STEVIE

WHO WAS SUCH A GOOD ASSISTANT
TO HIS DOCTOR

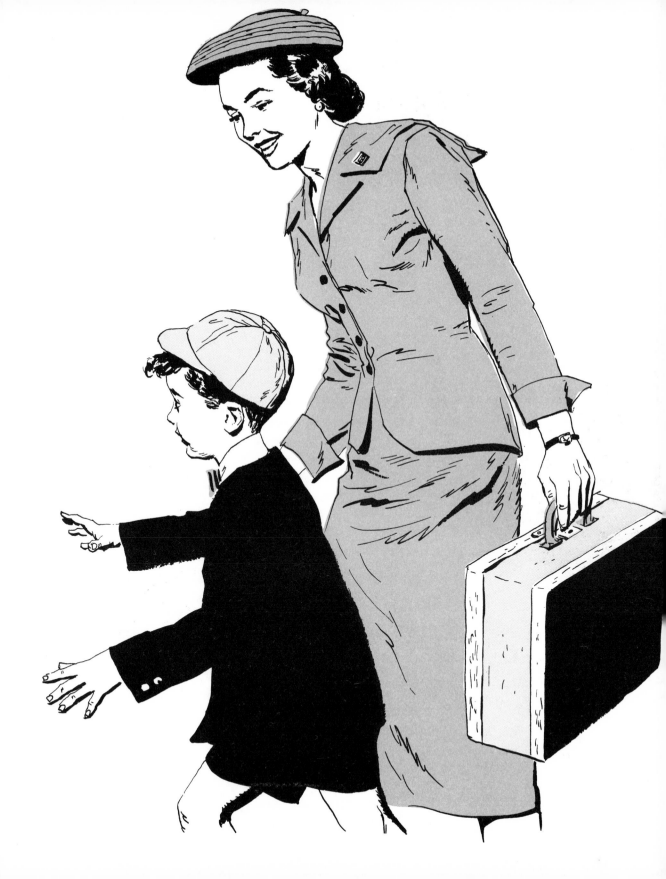

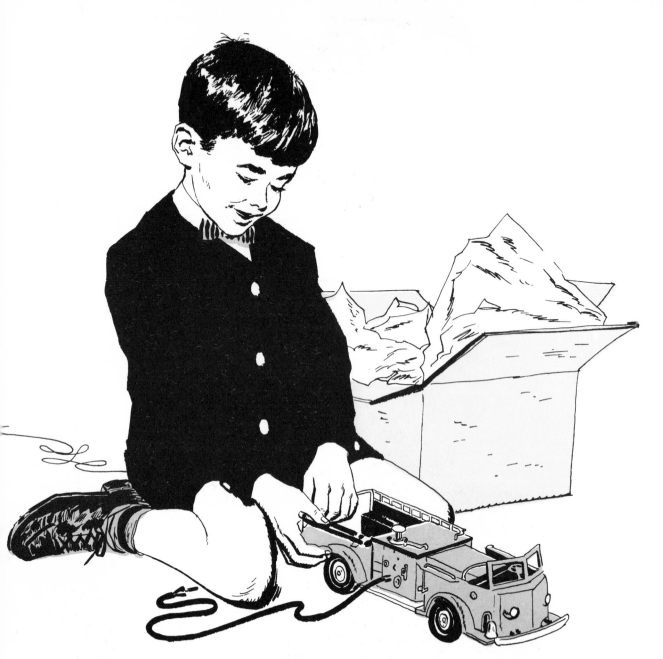

Stevie quickly opened the package. He couldn't wait to
see what was in it. It was a fire truck that squirted water—just
what he had wanted for so long!

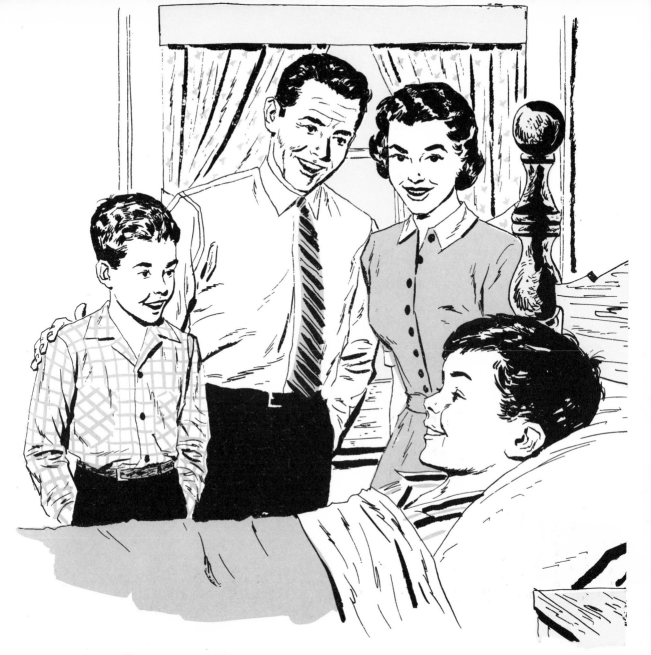

Stevie was tired. It felt good to get back in his own bed
again. He was glad his tonsil operation was all over.

Mommy, Daddy and Andy were so proud of Stevie. You
could tell that everybody was happy.

Are you going to the hospital to have an operation? Here are some of the things that you will probably see.

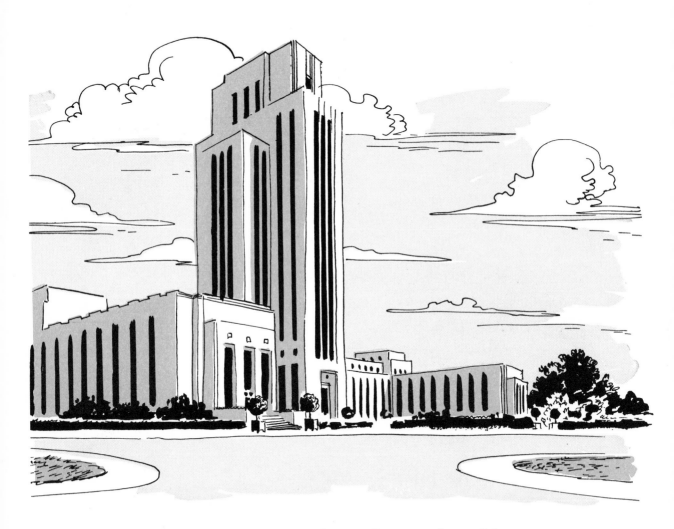

This is a hospital. Some hospitals are bigger than this—some are smaller. People take good care of you here.

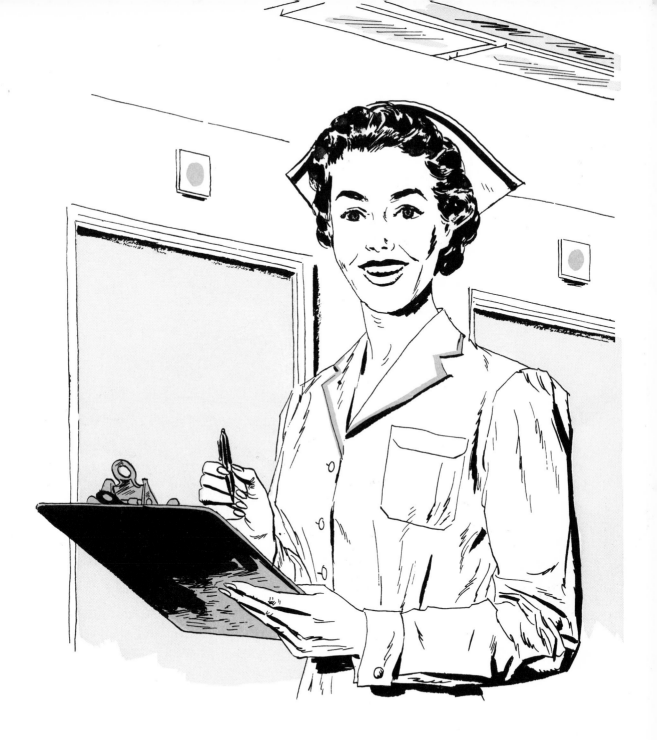

Here's one of the nurses in her spic-and-span white uniform. She'll help the doctor—and she'll help you, too!

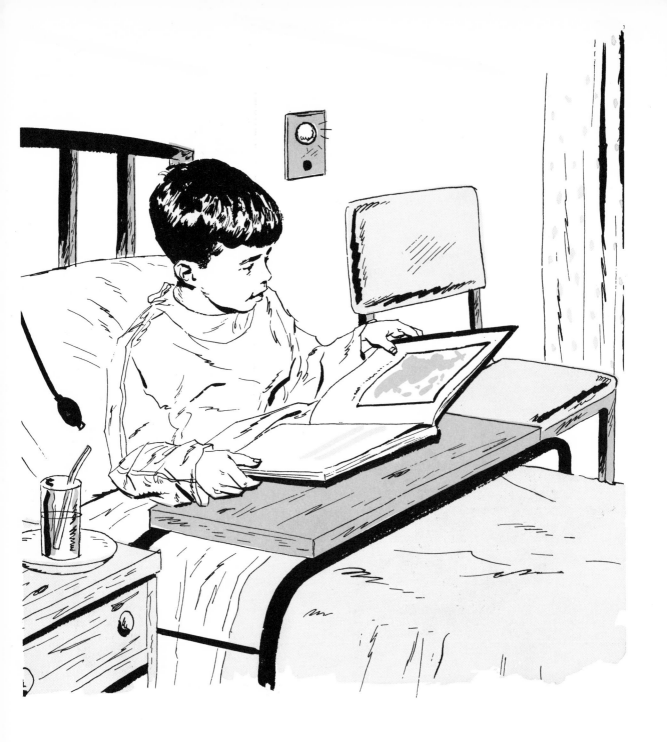

If you have your own room in the hospital, it may look like this.

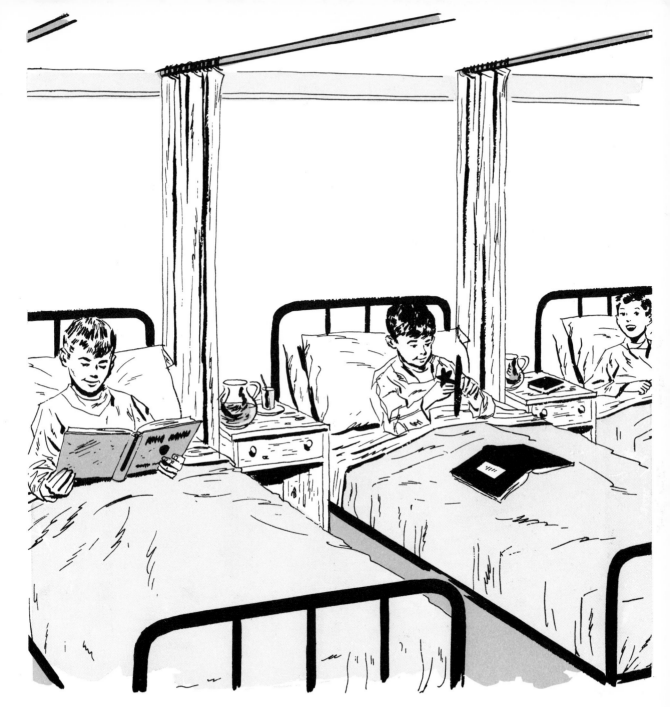

Or maybe you'll be in a big room with other children. You'll like eating on the tray that wheels over your bed. Curtains can be drawn between beds, too.

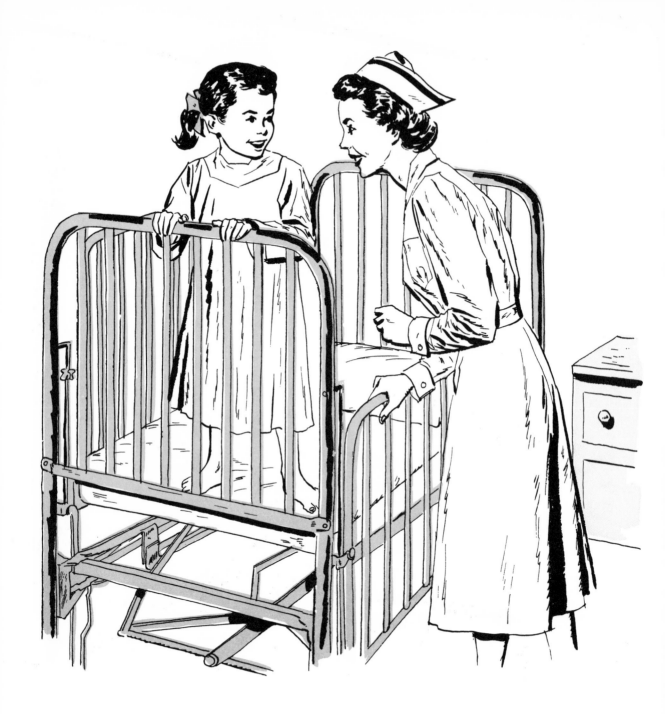

If you're not too old, your bed may be a big crib. Most children like it while they're in the hospital.

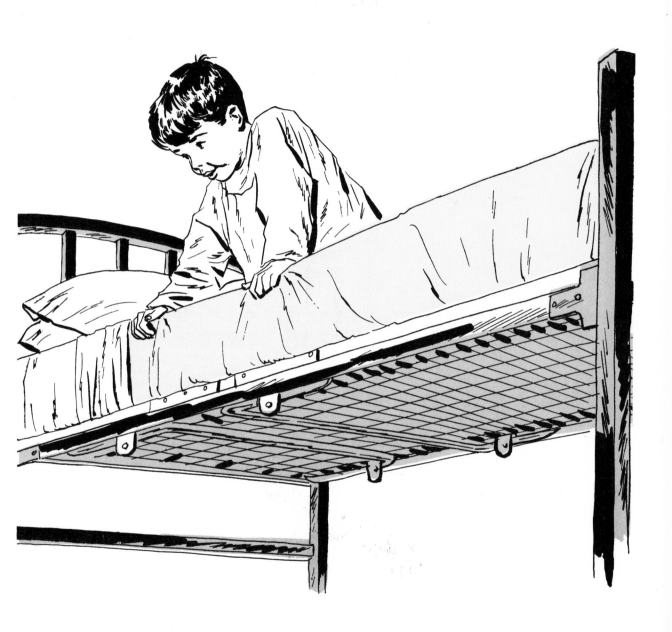

But if you have a hospital bed, it will look like this. It's higher than your bed at home so nurses can help you more easily.

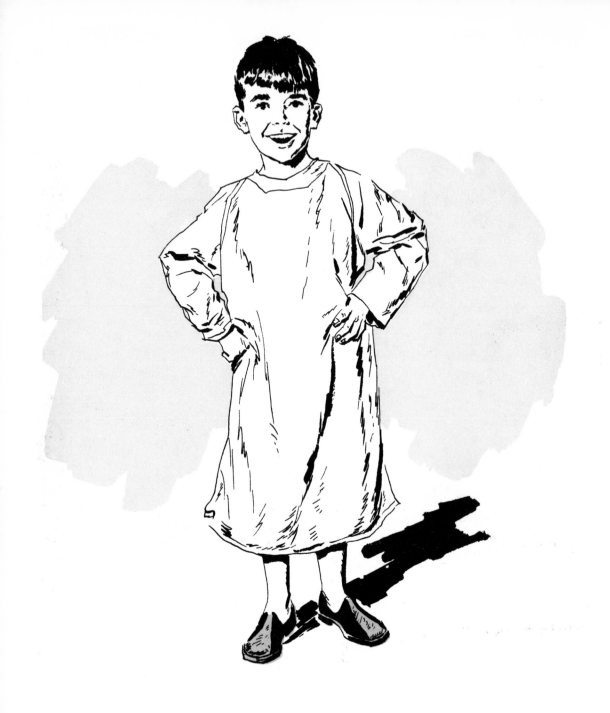

At the hospital, children wear a little white jacket instead of pajamas. It buttons in the back.

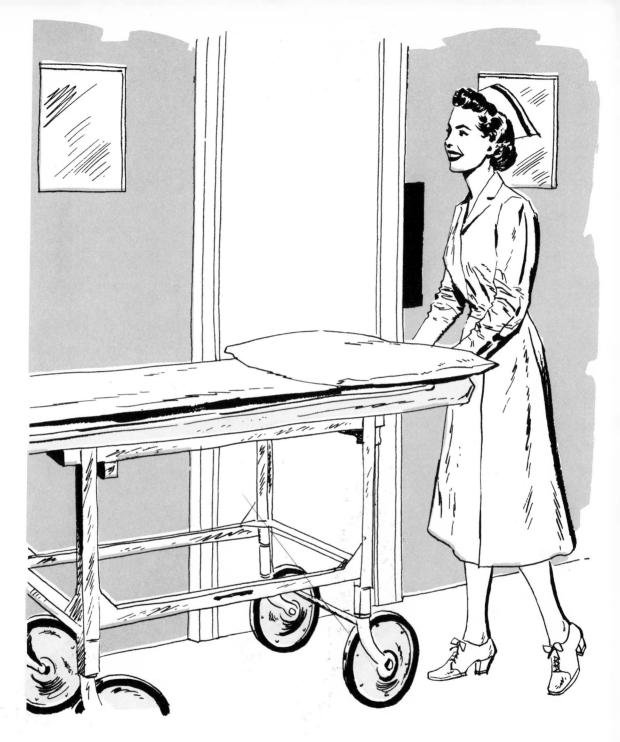

In some hospitals you have a ride to the operating room on one of these tables.

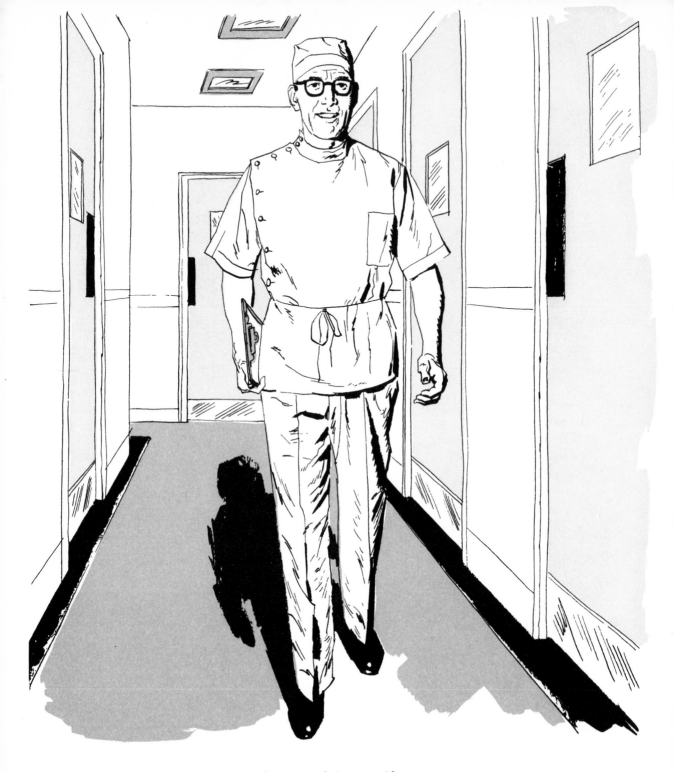

Here's the doctor in his clean, white uniform.

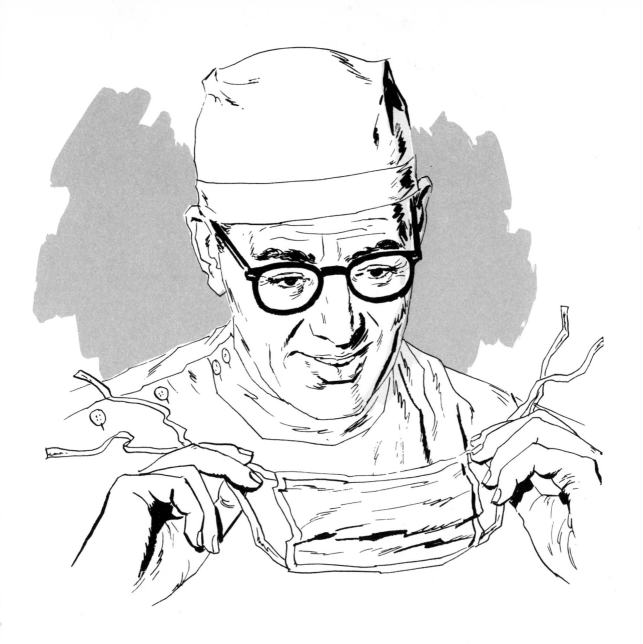

He'll wear a little mask over his nose and mouth in the operating room—so will the nurses.

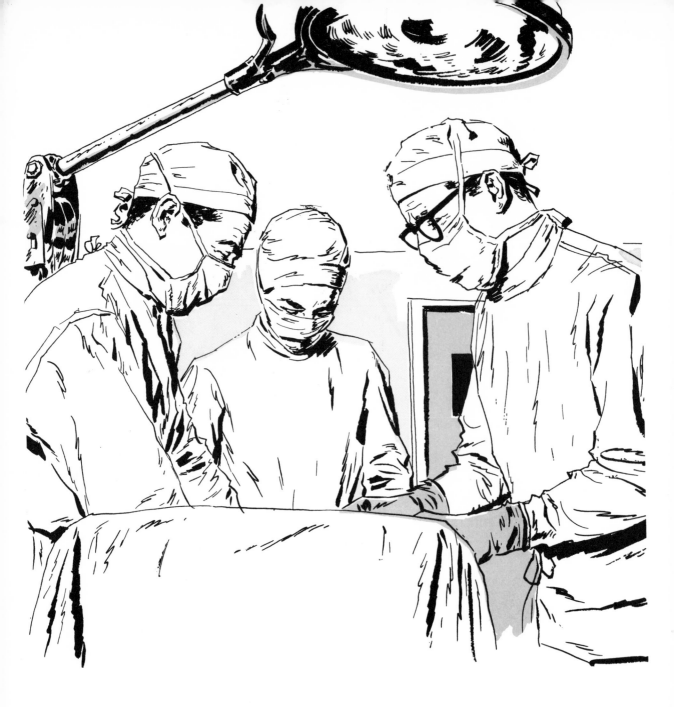

This is the operating room. You'll be here, fast asleep, until the
operation is finished.

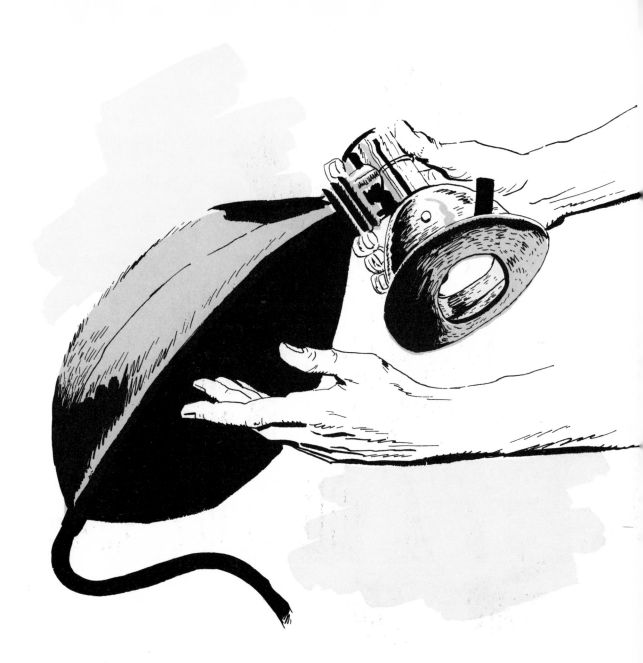

This is the balloon you blow into to fall fast asleep. You'll wake up when the operation is over.

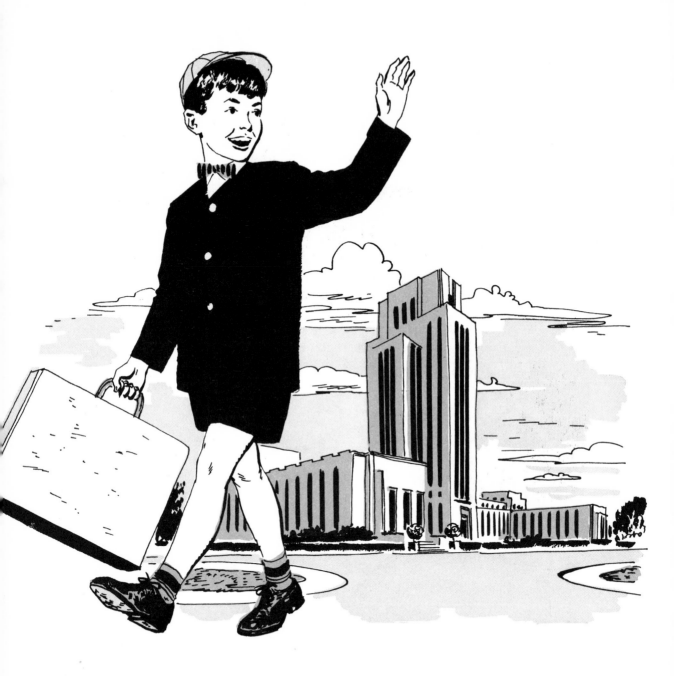

And now, pretend this is you leaving the hospital to go home!

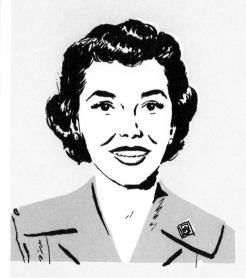
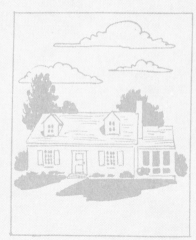
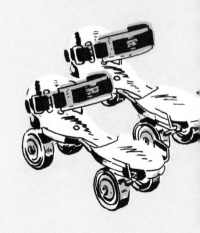
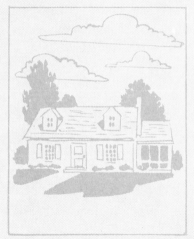
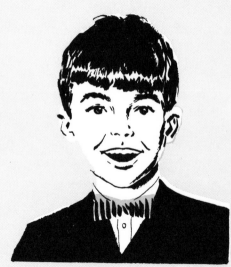
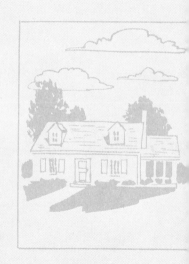
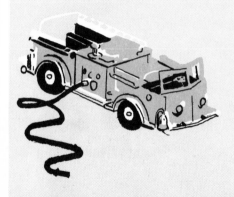
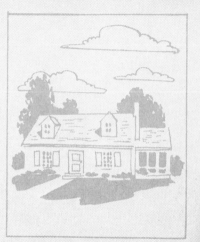
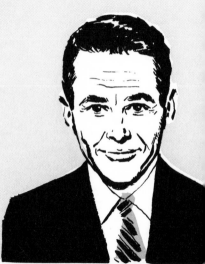

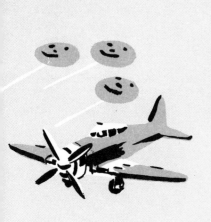
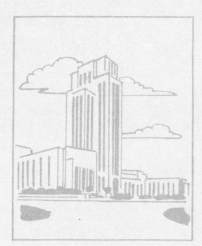
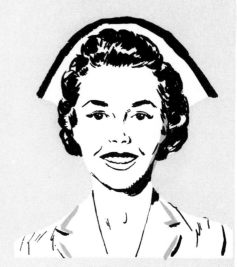
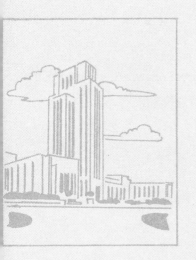
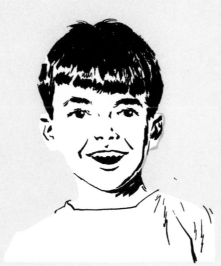
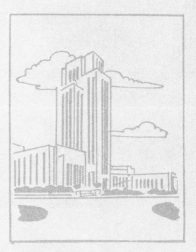
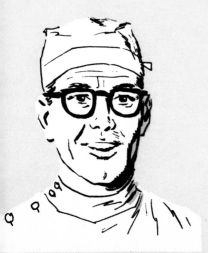
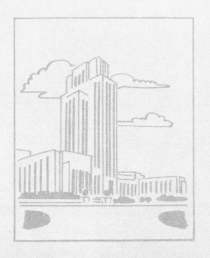
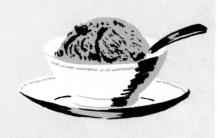